Optimum Health Secrets

Key Action Steps To Boost Your Energy

Tony J. Wilden

I0448038

TABLE OF CONTENTS

" You are what you breathe, drink, eat, think, feel, and do "

Tony Wilden

INTRODUCTION

Optimum Health Secrets is a unique book written by Tony J. Wilden who has been a natural healer since 1987. Tony is also a 5th Dan in Aikido and runs the Arun Aikido Club, which he founded in 1992 in West Sussex UK.

We hope you enjoy it and would love to have your valuable opinion at the Aikido Health Centre. Please visit - www.aikido-health.com/feedback.html

You can live a vibrant and healthy life by using the following tips every day... breathe deeply, drink pure water, eat organic food/supplements, focus on positive thoughts, relax, release your feelings, gently stretch for flexibility, list your life goals, and... take massive action on your plans.

" The art of healing comes from nature, not from the physician.

Therefore the physician must start from nature, with an open mind "

Paracelsus

" A journey of a thousand miles must begin with a single step "

Lao-Tzu

BEGIN YOUR JOURNEY TO

OPTIMUM HEALTH AND VITALITY...

AIR

YOU ARE WHAT YOU BREATHE

The first essential for life is air and the moment you cease to breathe your physical body begins to decay. Breathing is therefore the basic root of existence and must have prime consideration in any health problem.

There is only one correct method of healthy, natural breathing and that is deep, rhythmical inhalation and exhalation through the nose. It is essential to completely fill the lungs for optimum health benefits.

10-15 minutes of deep breathing upon rising and before retiring will be the most beneficial, but any time during the day will help you to alleviate any tension and aid the healing process within your body.

Have you noticed that mountain or sea air makes you feel a greater sense of well-being? This type of natural environment can promote healing, and it is surprising that we do not give more time and attention to it.

Of course, we don't all have the luxury of living near to a mountain or the sea, but you can use an 'air ionisers' in your home to help rebalance the negative and positive ions.

This can reduce any contaminants in your surrounding environment.

PURE AIR SUPPLIES OXYGEN AND VITAL ENERGY

There is a vital life force flowing through and around you, wanting to balance, heal, and give life. You must make its channels clear to allow it to do its work. This energy has been called magnetism, chi, ki, prana, etc.

You can tap into this energy and through special deep breathing techniques, you can gain more of this vital life force.

Whether you are studying healing arts, alternative Health, aikido or any spiritual path, there is ONE underlying core principle... **Attention on Correct Breathing!**

Yes now... breathe deeply and relax, YOU deserve it.

The time to relax is when you don't have time to!

In traditional Japanese arts, proper breathing is taught as an essential and fundamental factor of concentration. Oxygen contains energy and life from the universe, which your lungs receive through inhalation.

The life-force energy contained in the oxygen is transformed into human energy. Breathing in takes in supplies of vital life force and breathing out spreads this energy throughout your body.

And...

You can consciously learn to breathe more slowly, all you have to do is decide to spend time on it by taking Action... 5 or 6 deep, calm breaths per minute, with regular practise, will become a good habit, particularly while you sleep.

Deep breathing purifies your blood, reduces stress, and improves health.

YOU REQUIRE CLEAN AIR

We all regularly need to go out for a 'breath of fresh air', which relieves us from the stuffiness of an overheated or overcrowded room, but...

where can we find this fresh air?

Unfortunately, during this period of the earth's history, humankind have caused an imbalance in nature which is harmful to the planet's eco-system. This live-now and suffer-later attitude is creating problems for future generations...

our children, grandchildren, and great grandchildren.

Why does mountain or sea air make us feel good and promote healing? Why does the weather affect our mood? Why does an air-conditioned atmosphere feel 'dead'? The answer lies in its electrical state... its positive and negative ions.

In 1910 Albert Einstein and Conrad Harbicht took a Ph.D. thesis on why the mountain air of Davos was renowned for its health-giving properties. Their conclusion was that it was the 'air electricity'.

Ions are gas molecules that carry an electrical charge by gaining or losing an electron. In nature they are generated by ultra-violet light from the sun, lightning, and thunderstorms, the breaking of water by waves, waterfalls, mountain streams... even plants.

In our so-called 'modern lifestyle', we have created an environment that virtually eliminates negative ions from our atmosphere.

Pollution such as... car exhausts, air-conditioning, smoking, fluorescent lighting, electrical equipment, overcrowding, man-made fibre in clothes and carpets, all create positive ions that lead to poor health.

Unfortunately, there are also tons of chemicals used and pumped out by the manufacturing and food industries into our air, water, and food.

Negative ions are one of natures natural cleansers which aid in the destruction of airborne bacteria, and clears dust, pollen, allergens, smoke and other particles in the atmosphere.

These negative ions increase our capacity to take up oxygen and can improve our ability to deal with asthma, bronchitis, catarrh, the common cold, insomnia, migraine, eczema, headaches, tiredness, depression etc.

Where do we find these naturally occurring negative ions? Mountains, by the sea, lakes, forests, woods, etc. Yes, in large open spaces... nature!

Therefore many people are sick, ill, dis-eased and do not have a healthy lifestyle. We all tend to gather in towns that are overcrowded and breathe in the fumes in our environment... all in the name of progress!

CHANGE YOUR LIFE NOW BREATHE PURE AIR

You can protect yourself from the pollutants in the air by escaping regularly to breathe fresh air and good oxygen that is found in nature.

Go for a walk and find a place in nature away from the noise... a mountain, by the sea, a river or stream, in a forest or wood. Practise deep breathing, meditation, contemplation, and relaxation of mind and body.

When you leave behind the noise of a busy society, you can also leave behind your personal problems... just for while. This can have a rejuvenating effect on your attitude and can positively motivate you.

You can add to these powerful health benefits by opening the windows to your home and circulating fresh air into the living environment. Negative ion generators and air filtration units can be used in the home, office or car for those not fortunate enough to live near mountains, seas, waterfalls etc.

These simple and efficient steps will greatly improve your health and well-being.

" What lies behind us, and what lies before us

are tiny matters, compared to what lies within us "

Ralph Waldo Emerson

Knowledge is Power, but...

Action is the Key to Your Success - Breathe Deeply!

CONTINUE YOUR JOURNEY TO HEALTH...

WATER - YOU ARE WHAT YOU DRINK

Most of the planet is covered with water and the human body is 75%, so water is vital for good health. Nothing in the world can be compared to water for its weak and yielding nature that is, cleansing, purifying, and healing, but...

it also has great power and can be harmful.

Water, the second essential for life, transports nutrients and oxygen around your body, builds tissue and turns food into energy. It also collects waste material for removal via the kidneys, bladder and skin.

Every living cell requires fluid, air, and nutrients. And the purer it is, free from pollutants, and chemicals, the more toxins can be let into it for removal.

Normal adults excrete about two pints of water every 24 hours through the skin, two quarts through urination, one pint through the bowels, and one and quarter pints through the lungs by exhalation.

A healthy person should drink a minimum of an ounce of water for every pound of body weight, and at least double that in times of stress or illness.

Water refreshes the body, revitalises the vital organs, and raises the energy levels. Drinking enough can help prevent urine infections, kidney stones, and bladder cancer.

Studies suggest we should **drink about 2 litres daily** through drinks and food. We should also adjust our intake as required, when we use more energy through mental and physical activities etc.

Tea, coffee, and alcohol tend to cause dehydration, which can lead to tiredness, poor circulation, slow metabolism, high blood pressure, headaches, dizziness, aching joints, dry skin, poor immunity, stress, and weight gain.

So, it is essential to remove, or at least reduce them for a healthy lifestyle.

WATER THE BAD NEWS

Human and animal waste materials, agricultural fertilizers, pesticides, herbicides, and fungicides all cause contamination. 'Modern' industry causes serious pollution problems, as all public and industrial sewage eventually finds its way back to us, in our air, water, and food.

Where do all the life destroying chemicals that we pour down our sinks, toilets and drains actually end up? Millions of tons of poisonous material go from our homes each year to the rivers, and seas.

This water and its pollutants then find its way into our reservoirs and back into our tap water and food. Therefore it is so important to use biodegradable products that do not damage the environment.

The worst pollutants are the substances discharged as detergents, pesticides, petroleum, or other hydrocarbons... chemical substances that do not disolve in water but interact to form entirely new chemicals.

Also consider the network of old pipes that delivers water to your taps, and the variety of metals it picks up along the way, such as... iron, copper, brass, lead, chromium, fluoride, chlorine etc.

Inorganic substances can be harmful in small amounts: arsenic, lead, aluminum, mercury, copper, calcium, magnesium, iron etc.

These materials can accumulate in the body and may be related to problems with digestion, kidneys, arthritis, rheumatism, and hardening of the arteries.

Isn't it time for us to give top priority to cleaning up the mess in our own backyards. Perhaps 'they', the Governments, Industry, United Nations, etc. would tell us of the dangers... or would they?

Not if the profiteering must cease!

Cynical?

Maybe, but certainly realistic :)

New approaches to solving pollution problems are constantly presented but the cost and practicality stop implementation on a large scale. It now seems an impossible task of delivering pure water to our taps, so you'll have to take responsibility and choose to solve the problem within your own home.

INNER CLEANSING FOR HEALTH AND LONGEVITY

In the past few decades several water purification techniques, designed for home use, have been developed and used on a large scale. These often come down to your own personal choice...

Natural Mineral Water

Natural mineral water emerges from under the ground and flows over rocks before it is collected, which means it has a higher content of minerals. It must come from a protected source to be considered pollution free.

Spring Water

Spring water is collected directly from a spring that rises from the ground and must be filtered and bottled at the source. It must meet the same hygiene standards as natural mineral water.

Tap Water

Tap water comes from rivers, reservoirs and bore holes. It is treated to remove bacteria, heavy metals, pesticides and residue. It often contains chlorine and other disinfectant chemicals which may have undiscovered long-term effects on health. It is monitored to ensure it is within 'safety' limits.

Filtered Water

Water Filters - remove selected contaminants, usually through an activated charcoal filter, that must be replaced regularly. They do not remove nitrates, inorganic ions or bacteria. This relies on the effectiveness of the system, which must be carefully monitored.

Reverse Osmosis

Reverse Osmosis units' separate water from chemicals using a semi-permeable membrane. They don't remove micro-biological impurities and must be monitored closely. One of the most recommended methods available!

Distilled Water

Distillers simulate the natural cycle by boiling water to kill bacteria and leave contaminants behind. The steam is then condensed and collected for use. It is considered to be an effective method of purification, producing virtually pure H_2O. Some experts say it is good for detoxing, but not long-term use. This is because they believe it will attract and remove minerals from the body.

WHAT ARE YOUR OPTIONS?

Drink tap water and hope the government and the united nations will protect you. Drink bottled water which is available and expensive. Use a simple water filter jug that removes some of the toxins.

I recommend using a home water purification reverse osmosis system, and a water distiller for shorter periods. Distilled offers you 99.9% pure water.

Whatever your decision, water is essential to your life. It transports nutrients and oxygen around your body, builds tissue, and turns food into energy.

It refreshes your body, revitalizes your vital organs and raises your energy levels. You can improve your health by increasing the amount of pure water you drink.

Knowledge is Power, but Action is the Key to Your Success!

" We are what we repeatedly do. Excellence, then, is not an act, but a habit "

Aristotle

CONTINUE YOUR EXCITING JOURNEY TO HEALTH...

NUTRITION - YOU ARE WHAT YOU EAT

To live at your peak on planet earth, it is essential to develop a positive healthy lifestyle. As part of this lifestyle you must include a definite nutritional plan.

The foods and supplements you choose to eat daily can either improve your health or damage it...

the choice really is yours!

Positive health is not just an absence of disease but also an abundance of energy and vitality. This affects our mental and physical performance and can lead to a profound experience of clarity. well-being boosted energy levels, emotional balance, a sharp mind, and resistance to disease.

Today after a brief detour into science and inorganic medicines, humankind is once again being directed to the proper use of food to restore to abundant health a dis-ease ridden world. What you eat is...

directly related to how you think, feel, and act!

Your body is a marvelous factory that needs constant maintenance. Food provides the energy and essential nutrients for the body... carbohydrates, proteins, fats, vitamins, minerals, and trace elements.

A diet consisting of essential nerve-building vitamins, blood-building minerals, gland-stimulating protein, and hormone-nourishing unsaturated fatty acids will give you optimum nutrition and good health.

The correct balance of these nutrients is most important in preventing the development of illness, and dis-eases, some of which can be life threatening.

The normal body chemistry balance is approximately 80% alkaline and 20% acid.

It naturally follows that if you wish to maintain nature's chemical balance and enjoy the health, which results from it, you must make sure that your daily food intake is alkaline and that acid forming foods are reduced.

NUTRITION THE BAD NEWS

It is absolutely necessary to recognize the ill-effects of refining, processing, over-cooking and the convenience packaging of our foods. Food labels are often misleading and do not tell the whole story.

Your standard of life, how you act, think, and feel is directly related to the nutritional quality of your foods. Your body consists of the foods you eat and optimum health can only be built with pure nutrients.

One reason many people are tired is because the foods they choose to eat cannot be digested and absorbed. Instead it becomes waste matter that turns into toxins and poisons, causing dis-ease.

Today's farmers grow bumper crops of produce, their use of chemicals, pesticides and insecticides merely improves the appearance and increases the size of their yield.

An abundant harvest fails to compensate for nutrient depleted soil. Years of farming the same land has slowly drained the soil of essential minerals. Never has the human race been so well fed, yet nutrient starved.

 In the UK over 25 tonnes of pesticides are sprayed on crops every year. Exposure is linked to many health conditions... depression, poor memory, aggression, Parkinson's disease, asthma, eczema, migraine, bowel problems etc.

Governments allow pesticides because it is argued that they are safe to humans at low levels. These tests are only done on individual pesticides, and no-one has tested them in the infinite combinations we are forced to consume them in.

This all adds up to an untested chemical cocktail, and studies have shown they may be hundreds of times more toxic in combination than alone.

People who are young, elderly or stressed are more susceptible to toxins than the average healthy adult, so the set safety levels are meaningless.

You should aim to drastically reduce your exposure and intake of these chemicals by choosing organic foods as often as possible.

It is a good idea to look closely at the quality of the food you are eating. I recommend that all of your food should be natural, fresh and organically grown.

By supporting the organic movement back to nature, you are helping to reduce the damage of chemical pollution. This is a real threat to your health, your environment, and the future of humanity.

If you also use good quality organic supplements, then you can be sure to get all of the essential nutrients your mind, body and spirit needs to experience optimum health and well-being in your life... real health insurance!

" Healthy soil, healthy plants, healthy people "

Lady Eve Balfour - founder of The Soil Association, 1946

You can avoid consuming chemical cocktails that effect you, your family, and your environment, by choosing organically grown foods, which can...

vastly improve your health!

All organic foods and products grown or made in the UK must carry a 'Soil Association' certificate. This proves the safety and purity of the product.

NUTRITION THE KEY TO HEALTH

All the cells in your body are constantly changing - they grow, live, then die. The changeover of cells gives you the ability to regenerate healthy tissues, by changing your living and eating habits.

One of the secrets to recharging your energy is to gradually introduce raw organic fruits and vegetables, a pure source of nutrition, and full of essential goodness. Fruit is a natural cleanser and vegetables build and revitalize.

Raw foods are full of enzymes, vitamins, minerals, and trace elements that are essential for health and a long, rewarding life.

Enzymes are found in protein and offer a key to longevity as they aid in the digestion and absorption of food. Sun ripened raw fruits and vegetables, raw nuts and seeds, sprouted seeds, dried herbs will all give you more energy.

The Japanese people tend to eat a lot of raw fish, vegetables, and fruits which bring general good health. This type of diet can revitalize your entire system.

Yes, it is a bit more expensive, but in reality, organic food should be part of a healthy lifestyle and not seen as a luxury. Eating non-organic food will cost more in the long run for your health.

FOODS TO AVOID

Some of the worst foods available are... sugar, alcohol, coffee, tea, hydrogenated fats, excess animal fats, fried, burnt, browned food, and refined or processed food with additives.

ORGANIC FOODS TO EAT

Recommended are... raw vegetables, fruits, whole grains, nuts and seeds, beans, lentils. Drink at least 6 glasses of pure water, diluted juice, herb & fruit teas every day, and supplement with an organic Superfood.

NUTRITIONAL SUPPLEMENTS ARE LIFE INSURANCE

The personal care industry still does not understand that many man-made chemicals are not compatible with the human body's composition. Science and nature should work together as tomorrow's well-being is rooted in today's thoughtful preparation.

True life insurance and assurance is to provide the body with all of the nutrients it needs on a daily basis in order to function properly. You and your family have a variety of nutritional needs, and they are unlikely to all be met through food. To boost and increase Your intake of essential nutrients try...

Multi-vitamin/mineral supplements, Juicing to consume more fruit and veg, sprouting seeds for protein enzymes, water and air purification, regular exercise, good sleep, deep breathing and relaxation etc.

MAGIC MINERALS

Researchers have discovered that trace minerals are needed to properly maintain our health and are a critical requirement for life. These natural healing agents are present in such small quantities that supplies are easily exhausted.

Science has proven that these minerals are life itself, and without them our tissues and organs weaken and waste away.

There is no escaping the truth that all elements work together. A shortage of just one mineral can disrupt the harmony and balance of the body's systems. While there are many minerals, all of which are vital...

The 'Magic 14 minerals' rule and dominate over all others.

If you eat the proper foods and supplements containing these 14 minerals, you will also be feeding yourself with the lesser known trace elements...

Calcium, Phosphorus, Iron, Iodine, Sodium, Potassium, Magnesium, Copper, Sulphur, Silicon, Zinc, Manganese, Chlorine, and Fluorine.

" Optimum Nutrition is the medicine of the future "

" You can trace every sickness, every disease,

and every ailment to a mineral deficiency "

Dr. Linus Pauling - Twice Nobel Prize Winner

A deficiency of protein, fats, and carbohydrates is very rare. But a deficiency of vitamins, minerals, and essential fats is very common.

Many nutritionists believe that only 1 in 10 people receive sufficient for optimum health. The following list of diet tips may be helpful to consume daily...

1 - One heaped teaspoonful of ground seeds.

2 - Two servings of beans, lentils, quinoa, tofu (soya) or 'seed' vegetables.

3 - Three pieces of fresh fruit... apples, pears, bananas, berries, melons or citrus.

4 - Four servings of whole grains... rice, millet, rye, oats, corn, bread, or pasta.

5 - Five servings of dark green leaf or root vegetables... watercress, carrots, sweet potatoes, broccoli, spinach, green beans, peas, peppers, etc.

6 - Six glasses of water, diluted juices, herbal or fruit teas.

7 - Eat whole, organic raw food, as often as possible.

8 - Supplement an organic super-food green powder.

9 - Avoid fried, burnt, browned food, hydrogenated fats, and excess animal fat.

10 - Avoid any forms of sugar, and white, refined, or processed food with chemical additives, minimize your intake of alcohol, coffee, and tea.

Certain rays of the sun can only be taken into the body through eating chlorophyll and no-where else. It is a strange semi-chemical and spiritual essence in plants that gives leaves their green colour and supplies vitality.

Science has shown that green leafy vegetables contain a high level of essential nutrients. The popular term 'Eat Your Greens' is good advice.

Of course, organic and raw is best :)

Watercress, dandelion, celery, green lettuce, green peas, green beans, onions used raw and added to your diet will supply essential vitamins and minerals.

Many of these greens are available as organic and living foods, that come in powder form. These are excellent supplements to ensure you are absorbing the recommended nutrients.

Some of the benefits of optimizing your intake of nutrients are...

improved intelligence, memory and mood, increasing energy and resistance to stress, achieving peak physical performance, turning back the clock, beating cancer, fighting infections naturally, detoxing the body, defeating allergies etc.

The real cause of illness and disease lies in an imbalance of the blood cells that weaken the nerve energy and stops the glands from functioning correctly.

The proper energy supply for the blood can be supplied in three ways...

1 - Through deep breathing of fresh air.

2 - Through drinking plenty of pure water.

3 - Through eating natural organic food.

" When it comes to eating right and exercising,

there is no ' I will start tomorrow ' Tomorrow is disease "

V.L. Allineare

Knowledge is Power, but Action is the Key to Your Success...

Eat Pure Organic Food & Supplements!

CONTINUE YOUR FASCINATING JOURNEY TO HEALTH...

MIND POWER

YOU ARE WHAT YOU THINK

What is the Mind?

It is everything connected to your intellectual and psychological functions.

It is possible that you may be part of a large experiment and your mind is controlled and manipulated by powerful Governments and Corporations.

Vast amounts of money spent on advertising and marketing suggests that you are under a continuous threat of many subtle mind control techniques.

In reality, you are responsible for your own physical and mental health and must take control or be controlled. Once you have taken control of your thoughts through disciplined mind power, you will be free of subtle controlling techniques used in our civilised modern society today.

Thought takes form in action, so what you think about you become.

Your actions have a reaction upon your mind, so it is absolutely necessary to cultivate and develop a calm and peaceful mental attitude.

Freeing yourself from worry, tension and strong emotions like anger can be achieved by looking directly and consciously at the fear involved.

You can take control of the present moment...

breathe deeply, relax, release and let go of emotional feelings as they come up.

Remember times when you have felt totally relaxed, vibrant, alive, in touch with yourself and aware of the connection with your environment.

For most people, these times are too brief and an benefit soon fades.

When you are calm and relaxed it becomes much easier to focus, concentrate and achieve your goals.

The time to relax is when you don't think you have time to...

Right Now!

CLEAR YOUR MIND

There is a powerful knowledge and wisdom of yourself that is hidden deep within. This true inner knowledge can be found beneath the mask of education, cultural and social conditioning, and is your birthright, and true character.

In order to clear your mind you must stop your mental chatter and internal voice, where you'll soon discover that are governed by instinct.

Most people prefer security, predictability, and even boredom by functioning automatically and superficially. This type of mind organises itself according to established habits and is narrow and unbalanced.

Of course, that's not you... right?

Each of us feels intuitively that there is another dimension where we can get free of these limitations and experience success, health and happiness.

The intuitive mind is relaxed, agile, receptive, resourceful and lives in the present moment. It is attentive to nature and has the wisdom to be relaxed and at ease with anyone and in any situation.

The human mind is a bridge between the lower dimensions of the body and the upper dimensions of spirit. The natural ability of intuition is suffocated in our early training and education, but we can work on these negative mind-sets that create eternal suffering, stress, and dis-ease.

To use your mind effectively you must clear any mental baggage.

We can experience a lack of awareness that results in problems, difficulties, and misfortunes, or we can experience the present moment with relaxation that leads to harmony, health, and happiness.

CONTROL YOUR THOUGHTS

The idea of taking control of your own thoughts may appear to be an impossible task, but, it is of vital importance that will prove entirely possible with some persistent practice.

Thoughts lie at the heart of everything and your way of thinking greatly influences your every action. Each of your thoughts is like a seed that germinates, sprouts, grows, develops, and bears fruit.

The thoughts that are repetitive and fill your mind develop more and more power and your subconscious mind leads you to their realization. Optimistic and confident thoughts will create an environment that will attract positive events.

Doubt is one of the most powerful blocks to your success. The process of creation of an idea through to its realization in material terms must include confidence and total belief on the outcome.

Here are some positive suggestions you may wish to repeat during the day and at bedtime, mentally or out loud, whichever feels best. Don't forget that repetitions and perseverance are the most important factors for success.

Each of my thoughts has real power in my life.

Every day I feel positive, healthy, and happy.

Every day I help others to live in harmony.

You can add many more positive statements depending on your desired results. Be specific, repeat, and develop strong beliefs. Within three months of using these affirmations positive changes will be noticeable by those around you.

BREATHE DEEPLY, RELAX, AND CONTEMPLATE YOUR LIFE

To clear the mental chatter from your life you will find many of the answers written in your life history that unfolds in cycles.

Each of these cycles of life have a natural teacher to pass on the wisdom you need to function normally and successfully in a complex and complicated world.

Your main teachers during these natural cycles were and are... Mother, Father, Yourself, Society, and the Universe. You can examine your life and learn from your history, beliefs, conditioning and the role you play out each day.

An excellent exercise to clear this mental baggage is to keep a Personal Diary.

You can reveal who you are by recording... poems, dreams, conversations, memories, observations, thoughts, intuitions, confessions, drawings, quotations etc. You will soon discover your true self by being honest.

It can be beneficial to examine your individual personal Life History Blueprint...

10 Defining Moments

Make a list of the ten most important moments that have had the greatest influence on your life. Think about the results of these events in your life.

7 Critical Choices

Make a list of the seven most important decisions you have ever made in your life. Contemplate and think about the results of these choices and actions.

5 Pivotal People

Make a list of the five most influential people and why they are important in your life. This list will probably include you, your mother and your father etc.

THE SECRET LAW OF ATTRACTION FOR POSITIVE MIND POWER

Have you heard of 'The Secret'?

It's a powerful message that is spreading round the planet. It is based on the Law of Attraction that states that you become what you think about.

Whatever thoughts and feelings You focus on... you will become!

There are principles and laws of nature that can attract positive energy to you. You can speed up the process of transforming your mind by working directly with your subconscious... this is true mind power.

This idea has been around for centuries and is used by almost all successful people in life. If you want to be successful and reach your dreams, desires, and life goals, you have to apply the secret law of energy attraction in your life.

MIND POWER SUCCESS TIPS

1 - Make a list of your desired goals in order of importance.

2 - Imagine them complete and list, in detail, the necessary steps to get there.

3 - Read at least 3 times every day. Imagine, visualise and meditate on success.

4 - Be relaxed, open and flexible to the subtle signs of success opportunities.

5 - Take massive action towards your goals - the key to your success.

6 - Use bursts of energy with hard thinking, instant action, and honest effort.

Knowledge is Power, but Action is the Key to Your Success...

Think Positive Thoughts!

CONTINUE YOUR INCREDIBLE JOURNEY TO HEALTH...

RELAXATION

YOU ARE WHAT YOU FEEL

Doctors and physicians know that nervous problems of tension, anxiety, irritability, anger, and many other forms of extreme emotions stop you from being relaxed and at ease.

If you are not at ease, then in time you will experience dis-ease, which allows your mental and emotional energy to trickle away in a constant stream with the resulting wear and tear on your nervous system.

If you clench your fists, chew gum, drum repeatedly, frown, and generally express your mental states in physical action you are wasting your energy.

This can be seen in all aspects of society, people are too busy and leading complicated lives with artificial habits. This puts a drain on energy resources and effects quality of life, leading to dis-ease, illness, shortened lifespan.

It really is essential to arrange your lifestyle and become more sensitive to your individual needs. You must learn to respect your internal rhythm and remember the hours before midnight are the most valuable to replenish vital energy.

We all need quality sleep and relaxation!

You can determine what is natural by observing that you are energetic after sunrise and tired and passive after sunset. So, nature tells you to get up at sunrise and retire at sunset for maximum benefits.

If you have not built up reserves of energy then you can become weakened, tired and drained. Good sleep and relaxation will help build these reserves.

When your muscles and nerves are at rest your mind and body is calm and energy is stored for future use.

An example of this can be seen in the animal world and particularly the cat family. Cats are relaxed but ready for instant action followed by instant relaxation again, there is no tension or waste of energy.

Most people who have mastered the ability to relax are usually active, vibrant and full of energy. The difference is that they do not waste energy.

Every action, mental or physical, conscious or subconscious, uses up a certain amount of vital life-force energy.

SLEEP AND RELAXATION

Three levels of sleep are repeated in a cycle four or five times during a night. The first level is shallow sleep, during which time the heart beat drops, breathing becomes slow and regular and the body is liable to toss and turn.

This is followed by a period of deep sleep, when both muscles and brain are relaxed, growth hormones are released, and protein production is increased.

During this period the body is repairing itself and dead cells are replaced.

Next a period of sleep where electrical activity of the brain increases, and the breathing and heart beat become irregular. It is at this level that we dream, which is indicated by rapid eye movement (REM).

Rest and relaxation can be gained by lying immobile without sleeping.

We sleep apparently to dream.

Recent research has indicated that time spent dreaming, which normally occupies about two hours every night, is the most important period of sleep.

So, if you can't sleep do not worry, just rest and relax. It is likely that during the sleep you do get, your brain fulfills its dreaming requirements.

Most of us counter-act the benefits of deep relaxation and sleep by using soft mattresses, watching television and eating before retiring etc.

If You are using energy for digestion or processing thoughts, you are not using it to repair and recharge your vital life-force energy while you sleep.

When you have slept well, you awaken with renewed energy and have a more positive outlook on the day ahead. It is so important to develop correct sleep patterns to put you in harmony with nature, and the natural flow of vital energy.

CONTROL YOUR EMOTIONS

Your emotions need to flow continuously as you experience them.

If the heart is closed or blocked, you are unable to express yourself and life lacks intensity and passion. The five basic emotions from which all others originate are...

Fear, Anger, Sadness, Joy, and Compassion.

Fear is a useful emotion that puts you on your guard, intensifies your awareness and enables you to identify and deal with threats as they occur.

If out of balance, fear can lead to a general paranoia and chronic mistrust of people. Unexpressed fear tends to tense the muscles of the jaw, neck, lower back and raises the shoulders.

Anger is a reaction that protects your integrity when you feel personal boundaries have been crossed. When you feel 'invaded' anger is a way to say 'NO' to an injustice or violation.

Justified anger is immediate, clear and requires no explanation. The physical signs can be seen everywhere... tense jaws, clenched fists, stiff backs, raised voices, and blazing eyes.

Sadness is an emotional relaxation or release that occurs when your expectations are not fulfilled. Outward signs include long face, hunched back, slumped shoulders, feet dragging on the ground etc.

We conclude that to be happy we must avoid sadness, but this not the case, you must accept the inevitable disappointments in life.

Joy is an expansive energy of dynamic well-being that invigorates you, makes your eyes shine and puts a spring in your step. Joy cures, strengthens and restores confidence in what your inner life should be.

You no longer avoid the fear of the present by always wanting to be somewhere else, in another situation, in the past, or uncertain future.

Compassion is being able to feel what another person is feeling while remaining sufficiently detached to understand their needs and to know what to say and do. Gestures that come from deep within the heart are a tonic and natural form of release for the body.

BREATHE DEEPLY, RELAX COMPLETELY AND LET-GO OF STRESS AND TENSION

Relaxation is a release of mental and muscular tension, and the ability to put your mind and body in a passive state. When your body is completely relaxed you are able to calm and control your mind and its chaotic thoughts.

Your heart rate slows down and the cells of your body are revitalised.

You can learn how to instantly relax and restore your energy, anywhere, at anytime, in just a few minutes. By using the secret techniques of yoga developed by Indian and Tibetan masters and adepts.

Here's a quick and easy exercise for you to try...

Settle yourself in a comfortable position, sitting or lying down. Close your eyes and breathe deeply in through your nose and out through your mouth.

Contract and tense all your muscles for 1-3 seconds, then relax, release and just let-go. Repeat several times, feel the tension flow out through your heels to the depths of the earth.

To improve the benefits of this simple exercise...

Visualise and imagine yourself in your ideal relaxing environment... by the sea, a flowing river or stream, in a forest or wood, at the foot or peak of a mountain, waves breaking on the shore, a garden full of colour, scent of flowers etc.

Breathe in the pure air, healing colours and beauty of your surroundings, and allow this energy to spread throughout your body and mind. Then as you breathe out let the stress and tension flow out into the depths of the earth.

To boost the benefits of this simple routine...

Begin and end each relaxation session by gently stretching your body. This recharges and revitalizes your physical and mental energy.

Take the benefits of this routine further to finally achieve restful sleep and relaxation by including a daily exercise routine.

INSTANT RELAXATION

Instant Relaxation can be used anywhere and anytime in only a few minutes to protect you from stress and restore your energy levels.

Try the following exercise based entirely upon breathing technique...

Inhale and breathe in deeply, through your nose. Hold your in-breath for 5-10 seconds. Exhale and breathe out deeply, through your mouth. Hold your out-breathe for 3-5 seconds. Repeat the above exercise 3-5 times.

You now have an effective, but simple tool to apply anywhere and anytime.

" Learn to be silent. Let your quiet mind listen and observe "

Pythagorus

CONTINUE YOUR AMAZING JOURNEY TO HEALTH...

EXERCISE

YOU ARE WHAT YOU DO

Human beings in their original state of living, had an abundance of exercise out of doors and were compelled to find food, prepare it, raise crops, build houses and gather fuel to live in simple comfort.

As they became more 'civilised' they delegated certain duties to others and confined themselves to limited activities. Today many of us do practically no physical work, while others only do physical work.

Everyone should take some exercise daily as part of a healthy lifestyle. The normal healthy body is nourished if it is used. If not, it will become weakened, leading to illness and dis-ease.

Long walks away from the stress of modern society are excellent. The woods and forests, streams, rivers and beaches, over hills and mountains... The planet Earth and nature waits patiently for you to realise her amazing benefits.

WHAT IS EXERCISE?

Exercise is a process where the cells of the body are placed under controlled stress and stimulated to reach a degree of metabolic efficiency. It increases your vigour, strength and vitality.

The key to a good workout is oxygen intake and the goal is to increase your aerobic capacity, which is the amount of oxygen your body can process within a given time. This is related to your ability to breathe deeply which ensures oxygen is carried by the bloodstream throughout your body.

Most forms of exercise are good at stimulating body tissue but leave aside the strengthening of others. An efficient form of training will be one which reaches every cell of the body.

There are thousands of fitness systems but according to research done by the North American Space Agency (NASA) - the power of simple bouncing is the most complete system, declaring it to be THE most efficient form of exercise.

Aerobic rebounding (mini trampoline) vibrates every cell in the body.

It increases muscular strength and stimulates lymphatic elimination of cellular toxins and waste materials. It also increases skeletal strength and enhances learning ability and of course...

its great fun :)

Other great forms of exercise are walking, running, swimming, chi kung, tai chi, yoga, aikido, martial arts, etc.

The yoga adepts focus the mind on their training routines, using it in connection with their bodily movements. This increases the benefits as the supply of vital energy is drawn through the body with intention.

You should put life and interest into your workout and avoid listless mechanical training with your mind elsewhere. If you have fun and enjoy it you will obtain the maximum benefit.

EXERCISE TIPS FOR YOUR SUCCESS

As you perform your individual routine, there are certain simple techniques you can use to get the maximum benefits from the minimum amount of effort.

An effective and efficient plan will save you time.

Deep breathing is an essential part of a good routine.

Zen meditation, relaxation and deep breathing will deliver the quality and amount of oxygen to your body as you exercise to really benefit your health.

Drink plenty of water as part of your daily routine and take sips as you workout. Pure water flushes toxins from your body and is a vital part of a healthy lifestyle.

Focus your attention and concentration on what you are doing, and the benefits will multiply. This can be applied to whatever you are doing in life and develops will power, mind power, and discipline.

Develop a level of mental awareness for your surrounding environment. A relaxed awareness will allow you to tune-in and see negative events developing, giving you the chance to avoid them.

Before you work-out its important to breathe deeply, relax, loosen up, rotate your joints and warm-up before stretching all the major muscles of the body.

This avoids potential injuries.

To improve overall flexibility all stretching should be done slowly without bouncing. Hold the stretch for 10-30 seconds as you relax and breathe out. This will ensure you benefit your health and not injure it.

The best exercise routine for you is one that inspires you to put your mind and body to work... as one. This will also help you to relax and ideally be a form that can be practised in your environment, wherever you stand on the planet.

The ancient Chinese system of qi gong or chi kung is a natural way to balance and boost your energy centres (chakras). It involves deep breathing, complete relaxation, and a focused mind.

Aikido is a Japanese martial art based on non-violence and evasive movements. An excellent fitness workout for self defence. There are millions of practitioners across the globe... highly recommended.

" *The sum of the whole is this: walk and be happy; walk and be healthy. The best way to lengthen out our days is to walk steadily and with a purpose* "

Charles Dickens

CONTINUE YOUR UNIQUE JOURNEY TO HEALTH...

LIFE GOALS

ACTION PLAN

To become the person, you truly wish to be, it is essential that you take control of your mind and use it for your benefit.

92% of worries are unnecessary...

40% never happen

30% have already happened and cannot be changed

12% are needless about health

10% petty miscellaneous

and only 8% are genuine!

You are where you are and what you are because of the thoughts that dominate your mind. You become what you think about. Therefore, you should act as the person you wish to become and expect the best.

Don't surrender to the push and pull of circumstances...

Act not re-act!

Your life is in your hands, take control and start towards your goals now. Each day you can write another page in the story of your life.

Success is a progressive realisation of a worthy goal, so know what you want, dream it, and create it. Write down the 7 most important things for you to do in order of importance. Then work on them one-by-one until completed.

Whatever you vividly imagine, ardently desire, sincerely believe, and enthusiastically act upon... must inevitably come to pass.

PLAN YOUR WAY TO OPTIMUM HEALTH

What do you want from your time here on Planet Earth. You must have a clear idea of your dreams, desires, and life goals. The rewards of life come to those who do, not to those who merely read, talk, or day-dream.

Deciding that you want to achieve a certain result by the end of the year, is an example of goal setting. High performance people set goals, winners set goals, losers never set goals.

Achieving health, wealth, and happiness starts with having a dream. The dreams you have today are surely tomorrows realities. Dreaming is a type of visualisation with passion on the things that you really want to be, have or do.

Here is a little exercise from master motivator Peter Thompson...

Imagine walking into a room and meeting the 'you' of five years from now. What will you be wearing? Where will you be living? What will your lifestyle be like? What car will you be driving? Will you be running a business?

If so, how successful will you be? What will your net worth be?

You really only have three choices here about how the 'you of the future' will look... somewhere in between how you are now, and a depressed, broke and scruffy tramp. An exact clone of how you are now - absolutely nothing has changed in a decade. A happier, wealthier, healthier version of the...

'you of today'.

Ask yourself the following questions...

What do I need to achieve in the next 12 months to make my future dream a reality? What do I need to do in the next month to start myself on this journey? What can I do by next week to prepare myself for the journey?

What can I do today, or **right now,** to start this process off?

We need to dream, but this is not enough.

Dreams are too large to realise in one hit. Our minds are finite, and so all large projects must be broken down into bite-sized chunks otherwise we may become discouraged by the scale of the endeavour.

This is a 'secret' of successful people, each step is manageable, and can be completed in anything from a few hours to a few weeks.

Take a sheet of blank paper and write on the top...

This is what I want to achieve in the next 12 months.

Now put the numbers 1-7 down the left-hand side of the paper and write seven things you want to achieve over the next 12 months.

Dream, then break your dreams down into bite-sized chunks, then set weekly, monthly, yearly goals and act on them to move you closer to your goals.

GOAL PLANNING FOR YOUR SUCCESS

Visualize and calmly maintain the image of your goal, imagine, and feel it coming true. Create your own mental cinema where you can focus on the detailed image and different aspects of your desire. You should not allow your mind to wander aimlessly, your thoughts must be clear and precise.

Breathe deeply and relax. When you are calm and relaxed, it becomes easier to concentrate, focus, and achieve your goals. Liberate your natural talents and go with the flow for unlimited energy.

When it comes to problem solving we tend to get bogged down in the details and lose sight of our goal. If we focus our thoughts on solving the problem, whilst removing our own opinion... then we can come to a rational conclusion.

Looking at things more objectively, we can see the bigger picture.

Prepare Your list of Life Goals...

1 - Make a list of your desired goals in order of importance.

2 - Imagine them complete and list the necessary steps to get there.

3 - Start with your first goal and focus your mind on its realisation.

4 - Work through the steps, one-by-one until successful.

5 - Take massive action towards your goals.

6 - Change your approach until successful.

" Happiness is when what you think, what you say,

and what you do are in harmony "

Mahatma Gandhi

Knowledge is Power, But...

Action is the Key to Your Success

Write Your Life Blueprint!

YOUR JOURNEY TO HEALTH IS ABOUT TO MOVE INTO OVERDRIVE...

SPECIAL

HEALTH SECRET

This version of Optimum Health Secrets includes an extra special bonus!

Here's your opportunity to use this absolute gem of wisdom. But before I give it to you, I am going to take a few moments to explain why it is so powerful...

Don't miss this opportunity to

Boost Your Energy Fast and Experience Incredible Health!

The information in Optimum Health Secrets offers you the key to real health and well-being. Use any one of them and your health will improve. If you put them all together, in a holistic way, you will soon be experiencing glowing health.

You may have noticed, at the end of each chapter, I ask you to act.

Why?

Well, its great to get useful information, knowledge and wisdom. But you must take action on it to make positive changes in your life. If you don't, then the information stays in your head as a concept or idea but is not being used.

I act on my plans and am heading, full steam, towards my life goals.

I invite you to join me by taking massive action yourself. Carry out the instructions in this book and finally...

Reach for YOUR dreams, desires and life goals!

I have been studying, practising and teaching aikido and healing for 30+ years. In that time, I have made an intense study of the key principles involved. This has led me to a series of insights in many areas of my work.

I have learnt that the human mind has been trained to make simple things very complicated. If something is difficult to understand, then we have a valid reason (excuse) for not doing it... right?

Therefore it is so important not to overlook the obvious for more complex answers. The masters have always said that the answers are...

Hidden in the Open!

In fact, they are so close to us that we cannot see them.

Please don't make the mistake of overlooking the health secret that I am going to reveal to you here. It is something very special indeed, and, in my opinion... the single most important thing you can do to improve your health.

You won't find this information elsewhere, because it has been hidden from the public. In fact, it took me 7 or 8 years of study as a member of a secret society before this powerful method was fully revealed to me.

And I was totally shocked that I had not thought of it before!

No, I am not going to tell you which underground organisation I was a member of... that would be unfair of me. But as I am no longer a member, and haven't been for some time, I feel it is time to reveal this...

Absolute Gem of Wisdom!

If you do overlook it in search of a magic pill, potion, or product... good luck, because the search is going to be long and very disappointing!

HEALTH PRINCIPLES

There are dozens of health principles, and I have covered many of them in this book. For this great health secret, I am going to set it up with just 3 principles...

1 - The oxygen and life force energy from the air you breathe.

2 - The waste removal from the water you drink.

3 - The nutrients from the food you eat.

The power of this health secret takes place in every cell of your body. You see, the health of each individual cell is dictated by the balance of positive and negative vibrations and life force energy present.

This energy is often known as... vital life force, chi, ki, prana, magnetic energy etc... there are many names for the same thing.

The important thing to understand here is that you can greatly affect this process, and power up the energy in your body cells. It is a very simple thing to do and will have a massive effect on your health.

If you have been carrying out my recommendations in this book, then the next health secret will change your life forever.

Yes... it is that powerful!

Okay, you must be getting impatient by now, and just want me to tell you, right? I'm getting there, but there are a couple more things to tell you first ;)

WHY IS THIS HEALTH SECRET SO POWERFUL?

Many of us know that we are supposed to breathe very deeply to get more air in our lungs. Also, to exhale strongly to remove poisons.

The deeper the breath the more air we draw in, but if the lower part of the lungs are full of stale air, that has been there for a long time, then we cannot fill that area with fresh air.

The average person only breathes with the top part of their lungs. The stale air at the bottom becomes heavy, devitalised and leads people to feel sleepy, drowsy, nervous, weary, etc.

You can make a massive difference by taking control of certain processes that take place at the bottom of your lungs. This is where the negative blood cells receive their positive polarity, which turns them into a living magnetic cell.

A vitalised cell flows powerfully around your body to do its important work. Blood cells carry nutrients around your body and collect poisons to be removed.

A balance of positive and negative qualities allows these cells to do a better job.

The negative energy of each blood cell is full of nutrients received from the food you eat. It then goes to the bottom of the lungs to absorb the magnetic positive energy from the air.

It takes place through a thin membrane, in a process, technically called osmosis.

This is where things tend to go wrong!

There is not enough positive energy available and the blood cell remains out of balance. Positive and negative elements are always looking to attract the opposite to them...

yin-yang, hard-soft, male-female, positive-negative, etc.

The air you breathe is charged with vital life force, known in sacred writings as 'the breath of life'. This is the vital energy that flows throughout the universe and is the secret of the creation of life itself.

Through deep breathing you can fill your lungs with a vital life force that each blood cell desperately needs. The more negative energy the cell holds the more positive it can attract and absorb.

Weakened cells do a poor job which leads to illness and eventually dis-ease. Good food elements build better blood cells, which attract more vitality.

SPECIAL HEALTH SECRET

To get the very best effects from this #1 health secret you must...

1 - Breath deeply.

2 - Drink plenty of fresh, pure water.

3 - Eat organic food and supplements.

4 - Exercise regularly.

5 - Relax completely.

Okay everything is in place to finally tell you this unique health secret...

about time eh?

Just before I do, I must remind you that the secrets to life are hidden in the open. And that the most powerful principles are simple, easy-to-apply, and free!

Here is the Secret...

ADD MORE POSITIVE ENERGY

TO YOUR BLOOD CELLS THROUGH YOUR LUNGS!

Wow... is that it?

Well, I did tell you that the most powerful things in life are simple!

Please don't make the mistake of overlooking this in search of something more important... there just isn't anything more important to your health than this.

Do you agree?

Great!

You have just learnt **THE most powerful** thing you can do to improve your health. Of course, I won't leave it there.

After all, you want to know the very best way of doing this.

ADD MORE POSITIVE ENERGY TO YOUR BLOOD CELLS THROUGH YOUR LUNGS!

Of course, deep breathing is part of the answer. But, you must get fresh air to the bottom part of your lungs to get the very best effect.

The following method is easy to do and can be performed at any time of your day. If anyone notices and asks you what you are doing, then you can tell them the secret and help them improve their own health.

Please bear in mind that fresh air is best, so this method will not be so effective in... cities, towns, air-conditioned environments, poorly ventilated areas, etc.

Using an ioniser can help to purify the air but will not add vital life force energy.

Recommended places include... by the sea, lakes, rivers, in forests, woods, open spaces, mountains, hills, peaks, on ley lines (power spots around the globe), etc.

These are some of the best places to practise this secret method, but it is important to do it daily... regardless of conditions.

What is the Best Method of increasing the positive energy in your blood cells...

HOLD YOUR BREATH!

There is a contact healing system that I use based around this simple, but very powerful technique. Holding the breath gives you extra energy that can be transmitted to other people for healing purposes.

Of course, it takes a long time, focused study, and practise to develop this skill. But, if you just want to heal yourself... elements of it can be used much faster.

How can you do this?

First of all, please note that if you rush headlong into this practise you may harm yourself. This is because a sudden excess of oxygen can make you light-headed, dizzy, nauseous, etc.

Therefore you must build it up gradually and carefully.

NB: If you have a lung or heart condition, do not perform this breath-holding exercise. Just breathe deeply and get plenty of gentle exercise.

PLAN OF ACTION

1 - find a well-ventilated place (fresh air), where you wont be disturbed.

2 - get comfortable... stand, sit down, kneel, or cross-legged.

3 - take a few deep breaths and relax completely... let-go of any tension.

4 - perform this routine a maximum of 5 times in any one period (day).

5 - inhale slowly in through your nose and fill the bottom of your lungs by pushing your stomach out. Hold it for 10 seconds. Then exhale slowly by pulling your stomach in. Repeat up to 5 times, a few times a day for a week.

Don't overdo it!

6 - repeat tip 5 but increase the breath hold to 15 seconds on the second week, 20 seconds on the third week, and so on. In this way you will increase the breath hold by just 5 seconds per week. Try and increase it to 45-60 seconds.

Personally, I do more, in order to get excess energy for healing purposes. Eventually you can practise this method any time you like, wherever you are.

But don't overdo it!

THAT'S IT!

There is a lot more to it, but this is the essence.

By practising every day, you'll soon notice the difference. In time, you will feel a powerful energy that flows throughout your body.

In fact, other people will notice a massive change in you too!

Apart from releasing all those little health problems you may be experiencing, you may begin to feel like you can help other people with this technique.

If that is the case and you want to learn more about my **contact healing system** I will be preparing an ebook/book/mp3 audio. This is a very powerful healing method that you won't find elsewhere. Unfortunately, it's not available yet...

But it will be worth the wait :)

You can only make positive changes to your lifestyle by acting. If you just read this book and then move on to the next thing...

Nothing Will Change!

To make changes you must want it enough. Otherwise your motivation will reduce, and things return to how they were. You don't want that... do you?

The way to push through on lifestyle changes is to be inspired enough to take massive action, rather than motivated to do so.

Inspiration pulls you forwards, motivation pushes you forwards.

Inspiration

pulled magnetically forward - attracted like a magnet... Powerful!

Motivation

pushed, forced, acting against your will... Weak!

Okay that's it.

All that remains for me to say is...

best wishes for **YOUR Success!**

" You are what you breathe, drink, eat, think, feel, and do "

Tony Wilden

Breathe Deeply - Hold Your Breath...

ACTION IS THE

KEY TO YOUR SUCCESS!

OPTIMUM HEALTH SECRETS

SUMMARY

YOU ARE WHAT YOU BREATHE, DRINK, EAT, THINK, FEEL AND DO...

Breathe DEEPLY and Relax

Drink Plenty of PURE Water

Eat ORGANIC Food and Supplements

Focus on POSITIVE Thoughts

Positively EXPRESS Your Feelings

Gently STRETCH for Flexibility

List Your Life GOALS

ACT on Your Plans

" The art of medicine consists of amusing the patient

while nature cures the disease "

Voltaire

I hope YOU enjoyed reading my Optimum Health Secrets book and trust you will **Take Action** to improve your lifestyle. I welcome your comments and questions. Visit the Aikido Health Centre online... www.aikido-health.com/feedback.html

RESOURCES

Aikido Health Centre

Unique information on aikido, health, alternative health, well-being, spirituality, martial arts, self defence and much more. Visit... www.aikido-health.com

Harmony of Mind-Body-Spirit

Subscribe to our harmony ezine and receive free monthly editions straight to your email inbox. You'll also get some amazing free gifts. Remember to bookmark our email address. Visit... www.aikido-health.com/Ezine.html

Review This Product

Give us a positive and honest review of this book. In return for allowing us to use your testimonial on our site and in our promotions... you'll get a fantastic gift worth $47 Details at... www.aikido-health.com/testimonials.html

DISCLAIMER

Our intention, in Optimum Health Secrets, is to supply useful information to help you take control of your own health. Please use this with the advice of your health care advisor for total peace of mind. Knowledge is power, but...

Action is the Key to Your Success!

www.ingramcontent.com/pod-product-compliance
Lightning Source LLC
Chambersburg PA
CBHW070404290526
45790CB00004B/1633